INSOMNIA : ITS CAUSES AND CURE.

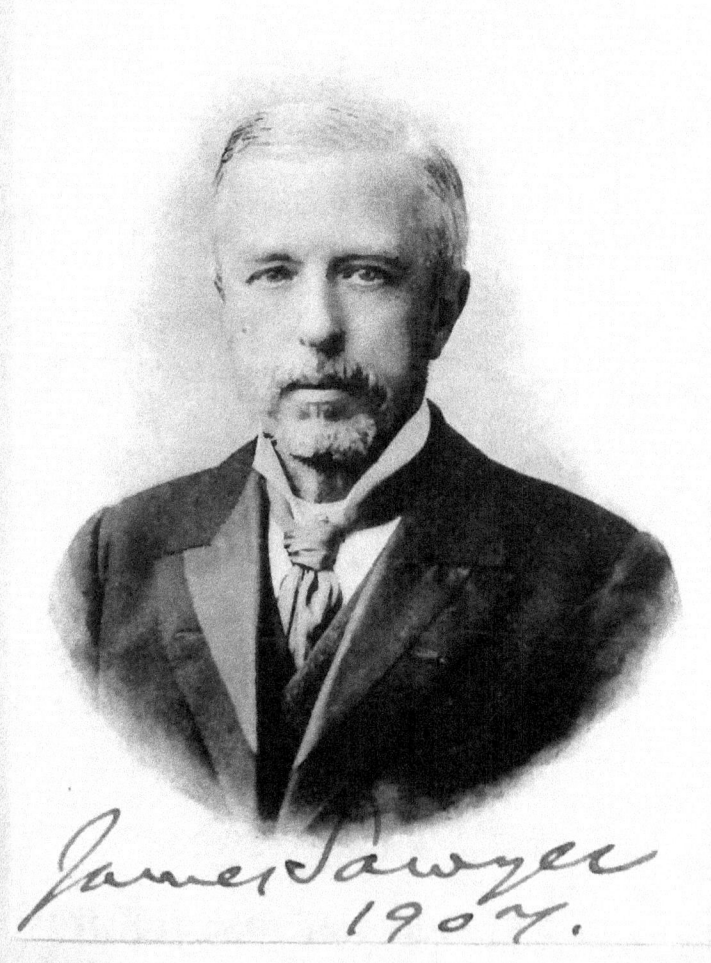

James Sawyer
1907.

INSOMNIA:

ITS CAUSES AND CURE.

BY

JAMES SAWYER,

SENIOR CONSULTING PHYSICIAN TO THE QUEEN'S
HOSPITAL, BIRMINGHAM.

Birmingham:
CORNISH BROS.,
1904.

PREFACE.

The following pages are the first two of the chapters of "Contributions to Practical Medicine," as they stand in the fourth edition, 1904, of that book. They include my lectures on the causes and treatment of insomnia, in the necessarily colloquial style in which they were uttered. For the convenience of my professional brethren, these chapters now are offered to them in a separate form in this little book. Every word has been revised and many additions have been made, by the fruits of later experience, for the sake of clearness, completeness, and precision; this has been done with hope of usefulness in medical practice, and with the aim of accuracy in diagnosis and success in therapeutics.

31, TEMPLE ROW,
    BIRMINGHAM, 1904.

CONTENTS.

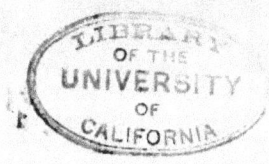

I.

THE CAUSES OF INSOMNIA.*

*The appetite of sleep.—The Physiology of sleep.—
Etiology of insomnia.—Symptomatic insomnia.—Intrinsic insomnia.—Varieties of
intrinsic insomnia. — Psychic insomnia.—
Emotional shock and prolonged mental
strain as causes of insomnia.—The nervous
temperament.—Symptoms of intrinsic insomnia. — Toxic insomnia. — Insomnia from
tobacco.—Alcoholic insomnia.—Insomnia from
tea or from coffee. — Gouty insomnia.—
Senile insomnia.*

THE important subject of insomnia has engaged
my attention for a long time. In 1878 I delivered a clinical lecture on the causes and cure
of insomnia to the students of the Birmingham
Medical School, in the Queen's Hospital, and
the matter of this discourse was afterwards

---

* A Clinical Lecture : published in *The British Medical
Journal*, December 1st, 1900 ; lately revised, rewritten, and
extended.

further published in *The Lancet*, on June 15th
and 22nd of that year. This lecture I revised
and rewrote entirely afterwards, embodying
in it some additions from my later experience
in practice, and, so enlarged, it was included
in each of the two editions, of 1886 and 1891,
of my "Contributions to Practical Medicine."
In the autumn of the year 1900, I reviewed the
subject again in two clinical lectures which I
gave at my hospital, and these were issued in
print in *The British Medical Journal*, on
December 1st and 8th, 1900. These last lectures,
in which I have tried to bring their subject up
to a point at least abreast of our latest knowledge in the principles and practice of medicine,
I have revised and rewritten; and I have
amplified them, especially in their therapeutic
parts. So rewrought, they form the contents
of the following essay. This work, done as
to the causes and cure of insomnia, that is,
done as to particular diagnostic and therapeutic
efforts in which the skill of the physician and
the resources of our art are often taxed severely,
in the intricacies of a difficult, delicate, and
abstruse subject, I have tried to accomplish in
the spirit of the Baconian philosophy, in the
spirit of that aphorism of Bacon which Sydenham prefixed to his renowned "Tractatus de

Podagra et Hydrope," namely, "Non fingen-
dum aut excogitandum, sed inveniendum,
quid Natura faciat, aut ferat." The result of
my pleasant labours I venture now to offer
to the judgment of my profession. My lectures
on insomnia were delivered for the instruction
of medical students in my clinical class; they
are further published in these pages in the hope
that they may help my medical readers in
practice. In view of the conditions of the
original delivery of these utterances, I have
decided, in revising them, to preserve their
colloquial style. Furthermore, in preparation
for this present publication of these lectures,
(1904,) I have revised them again, and made
some additions to the therapeutics of my
subject.

Sleep is a function of life, and life, in
some sense, may be said to be a function
of sleep, in man, in the animals which are a
little lower than he is, in some sort in plants,
in everything which lives. The living organism
which cannot sleep cannot live. For all beings
endowed with the crowning mercy of consciousness sleep is a pleasure as well as an appetite, and it is a necessity as well as both. For
these conscious beings, strung as they are in
their sentience to the most exquisite responses

in the world's vast chorus of living harmonies, sleep is indeed and in truth "tired nature's sweet restorer." For man, at the head of such beings, and perhaps the only of them which knows the cark of a mind's unrepose, or the wear of "that unrest which men miscall delight," sleep it is indeed which smoothes out life's fretting creases and "knits up the ravelled sleeve of care." That you may become practitioners of medicine you are students in this place of the manifold sciences of medicine in some of their chief practical bearings, mingled with the inexorable simplicities and with the endless intricacies of the art of healing. You are clinical students here of that cherished art of ours, an art which is of men philanthropic and of time perennial, as its lovely figure stands revealed in all its subtle and splendid details, firm and broad based upon the blended foundations of its great constituent sciences. You are students in this hospital I love of that great art of ours in clinical medicine, in its concrete application to individual cases of human suffering, no two of them indeed ever quite identical, no more than are identical a tree's waving leaves or the billows of the rolling sea. Let us press forward together, in all the absorbing zest of the pursuit which is ours, to the brightest understanding which yet there may be of the intimate nature of sleep. Let us collect, discriminate and sort the causes which make for insomnia. Let us sift and sum up all which our sciences and our art, our experience, and even our empiricism, of which last I am not ashamed, have of tried adoption for its cure. In this work your physiological training, your clinical insight, your utilitarian aim, and even your poetic fancy and your literary culture, may all find coördinated play, in the comprehension and in the verbal depiction of functions and maladies which are intricate with our lives, associate with our highest attributes, and woven in woof and warp into the very texture of all our pains and of all our pleasures.

Favoured by your kind attention, I purpose to offer you some considerations upon the vital function of sleep, and upon the conditions, causes, and cure of insomnia, based upon a somewhat long and successful experience of those subjects in practice, as a physician. These subjects are certainly of first-rate importance in relation to our knowledge of the science and our practice of the art of medicine. Possibly you may scarcely be able to appreciate their relative importance while you are, as yet, only hospital students. Later in your careers, when you become engaged in actual practice among the sick, and especially when you take part in what is called private practice, often will you be confronted by the perplexities of insomnia, and often will your pleasant duty lie in successfully unravelling the causes of sleeplessness, on that soundest principle of causation and of therapeutics, *cessante causâ cessat et effectus*, and in curing insomnia by counteracting those causes, and by making their tiresome and diresome effects to cease. I hope to be able to show you that in such happy results the science and the art of the physician may play a successful part. Like thirst and like hunger, sleep is an appetite. We may define an appetite, in the words of the philosopher Bain, to be a craving produced by the recurring wants and necessities of our bodily or organic life.* An appetite, strictly so-called, has two characteristic marks, and these marks are strikingly characteristic of sleep; these marks are two conditions which are true to sleep—namely, its periodic recurrence and its organic necessity. We know that the natural course of a human life brings on sleep without the volition of the individual willing the event. The true character of sleep as a

---

* The Senses and the Intellect.

veritable appetite appears when it is resisted. Under such resistance the individual person experiences what is called, in metaphysical parlance, a "massive" form of uneasiness, discomfort, and pain. The will of the individual, in the presence of this uneasiness, is energetically urged to remove such discomfort and unrest, and is urged from pain towards pleasure, is urged to obtain the gratification of relief in what Bain called "the corresponding voluminous pleasure of falling asleep."* In this imperatively urgent volitional impulse is the appetite of sleep. Sleep is a desire; with the further characteristics of its organic necessity, and its periodic recurrence, it ranks as one of our appetites.

The intimate physiology of sleep is a difficult subject, and the difficulties of its explanations have been the topics of much controversy, and such controversy appears to have issued from various combinations of the teachings of observation, of experiment, and of analogical and other reasoning, upon the phenomena of sleep. I do not propose to follow at length the details of this part of our subject. As a clinical teacher I must not overload your memories, but rather

* Mental and Moral Science.

must I try to make easy your mental digestion.
For our practical purposes I think we may
understand that two distinct, but associated
and related, vital changes occur in sleep. The
one is some intrinsic change in those ultimate
tissue elements of the brain which are concerned in consciousness; the other and
"coarser" change is a diminished supply of
blood to the brain, and especially to the blood
vessels of the cortex of that organ. The former
change is at present undemonstrable, excepting
by inferential reasoning. Perhaps there is some
essential and intrinsic change in the brain, and
perhaps there also is some such change in the
spinal cord and ganglionic nervous system, both
of rhythmic occurrence, and both conditions
of healthy sleep. Perhaps there is a functional
depression of these parts in sleep, and especially
of the cerebral cells, arising from "an accumulation in and around them," as Sir Thomas
Lauder Brunton puts the matter as to the
cerebral cells in sleep, of some of the products
of normal tissue waste. Perhaps for normal
sleep an intrinsic change of this kind must
gain the wide distribution I have mentioned.
It is likely that there is in sleep a rhythmic
change such as I have indicated, and that this
change is sustained by the physiological effects

of some of the issuants of those tissue changes, muscular and nervous, which especially occur in the active waking state of the body.

Perhaps for our sleep we must drown our cerebral cells in a kind of auto-intoxication with the ashes of our waking fires. We may usefully recall this view of the subject when we use exercise and fatigue as remedies for insomnia. The proof of the other broad change in sleep— namely, diminished blood supply to the brain, and especially to its cortex, rests on inference from physiological analogies, on various observations, and on the solid basis of direct experimental evidence. We must note, however, that the human brain, in its perceptive, cogitative, and volitional functions, in these great divisions of consciousness, is not the only part which sleeps. The whole living body sleeps. The changes which the event of sleep declares certainly extend beyond mere loss of consciousness; they extend to secretion, to the action of the heart and blood vessels in the general circulation of the blood, to respiration, to "reflexes," and so extend to all the tissue modifications, and to all the other vital activities, upon which such manifold transitions depend. In order to complete your precognitions of the physiology of sleep, before we pass on to consider the several conditions of insomnia and their appropriate therapeutics, I may refer your attention to the admirable accounts of these subjects to be found in the text-books of Dr. Augustus Waller* and of Sir Michael Foster.† From each of these volumes I offer a brief quotation, which sufficiently illustrates our subject for my present purpose. On that part of his subject which is so important to us from a therapeutical standpoint —namely, the state of the cerebral circulation during sleep, Dr. Waller says:

"Although there is no doubt that in coma —a pathological state similar in some respects to physiological sleep—the cerebral vessels are congested, the observations of Durham on the exposed cerebrum of sleeping dogs, and of Jackson on the retinal vessels of sleeping infants, are to the effect that vessels shrink in sleep, and we may therefore feel reasonably assured that the sleeping brain, in common with other resting organs, receives less blood than in its state of activity. Moreover, Mosso's investigations on exposed human brains afford

---

* An Introduction to Human Physiology. By Augustus D. Waller, M.D., F.R.S., 2nd Edition. London, 1893.

† A Text-Book of Physiology. By M. Foster, M.A., M.D., LL.D., F.R.S., 5th Edition, Part IV. London, 1891.

evidence that the organ becomes more vascular during mental activity...."

That sleep concerns the whole body, and not the brain alone, is well put by Sir Michael Foster. He says:

" Though the phenomena of sleep are largely confined to the central nervous system, and especially to the cerebral hemispheres, the whole body shares in the condition. The pulse and breathing are slower; the intestine, the bladder, and other internal muscular mechanisms are more or less at rest, and the secreting organs are less active, some apparently being wholly quiescent; the secretion of mucus attending a nasal catarrh is largely diminished during slumber, and the sleeper on waking rubs his eyes to bring back to his conjunctiva the needed moisture. The output of carbonic acid, and the intake of oxygen, especially the former, is lessened; the urine is less abundant, and the urea falls. Indeed, the whole metabolism and the dependent temperature of the body are lowered; but we cannot say at present how far these are the indirect results of the condition of the nervous system, or how far they indicate a partial slumbering of the several tissues."

You may find an interesting and instructive employment if you follow Sir Michael Foster through his discussion of the exact state of the body, and especially of the brain, in sleep. He points out, what is now generally accepted, that an alteration of the cerebral circulation is not the whole of sleep. He judges that " the essence of the condition is rather to be sought in purely molecular changes," and then he goes on to suggest a resemblance between the systole and diastole of the heart and the sleeping and waking of the brain; and then he dwells on the various periodicities which may be observed in the activities of the human body, and even suggests that the fundamental rhythm of the heart may be a reflection of the mysterious cycles of the universe, while it may yet be only the result of the inherent vibrations of the molecules of its own proper structure.

If we exclude from our consideration the insomnia which is a concomitant of some forms of unsoundness of mind, and which kind of insomnia I do not propose to deal with in these lectures, you will find that absent or imperfect sleep, inability to sleep at all, or at a convenient time, or long enough, without the aid of drugs, is a frequent consequence or complication of numerous and varied conditions of disease. Etilogy, as you know, is that division of the science of medicine which has to do with the

causes of disease. The etiology of insomnia
embraces the enumeration of all the causes of
the malady. These causes are numerous, and a
classification of the varieties of insomnia, upon
the basis of their causal distinctions, is somewhat difficult. Let me recommend to you, for
use in practice, the following classification of
the varieties of sleeplessness under our consideration. It is the best etiological arrange-
ment I can form, of the causal intricacies of
our subject. It is a classification which you
will find of service clinically, when you pursue
the discovery of the particular causation of any
given case of sleeplessness. Cases of insomnia
seem to divide themselves naturally into two
groups, namely, of cases of what may be called
symptomatic insomnia, and of cases of what
may be called *intrinsic insomnia*. Symptomatic
insomnia attends a vast variety of morbid
states, and is secondary to them, or is part of
them. Intrinsic insomnia, as we shall see later
on, is capable of distinct definition, and it
breaks up naturally and simply into three
smaller divisions, upon a causal principle of
division.

As to symptomatic insomnia, pain, if
severe enough, and from whatever cause
arising; pyrexial elevation of temperature;

frequent coughing, such as often occurs in pulmonary consumption; dyspnœa, such, for instance, as results from obstructive dilatation of the cardiac cavities, and appears to require an extraordinary vigilance of the nervous centres for the maintenance of the vital processes of respiration and circulation—are clinical conditions of disease which may prevent, shorten, or break up sleep. Such conditions are frequently met with in medical practice, as single causes of insomnia, or as conjoint causes of it in various combinations. In such and in similar instances the cause of the sleeplessness is obvious, and the consequential character of the insomnia—that is, its dependence upon a distinct and sufficient cause—is clear. For the therapeutic control of this kind of insomnia we may employ with success one of two curative methods, or we may employ a judicious combination of these methods, such combination being founded upon a skilled appreciation of the especial needs of each individual case. We may control sleeplessness of the kind in question either by the exhibition of remedies which directly cause sleep, that is to say, by the administration of some of the drugs which we know as hypnotics or soporifics, or we may control it by the employment of measures

which combat the cause of the insomnia, by
removing pain, by reducing the heat of fever,
by quelling cough, by relieving cardiac dis-
turbance and dyspnœal discomfort, and so on;
or by using in conjunction hypnotics and
remedies addressed to the removal of the cause
of the sleeplessness. In such cases of symptomatic insomnia, as in medical practice
generally, you will find that it is convenient
to your duties, and that it tends to the
thoroughness of your ministrations, if you
regard the therapeutic indications of each case
from the well-known standpoints, respectively,
of the *indicatio causalis,* of the *indicatio morbi,*
and of the *indicatio symptomatica.* By a
judicious combination of the remedies so suggested you will be able to deal successfully with
cases of symptomatic insomnia. By regarding
the cause of the illness with which you have to
deal as a medical attendant, by regarding the
various pathological processes which underlie
the progress of that illness, and by regarding
the symptoms of that illness, by regarding these
points in turn, or together, or in various combinations, with a judicious therapeutic inten-
tion, you may arrange your remedial efforts
upon a systematic and comprehensive basis.

Now let us consider the details of intrinsic

insomnia. There is a simple inability to sleep,
which you will often be required to cure—a
kind of insomnia which may be called for the
sake of simplicity, but perhaps scarcely with
strict truth, *insomnia per se*. This is a kind of
wakefulnes for which we cannot discover an
objective or obvious physical cause; it is a kind
of wakefulness which seems to depend upon an
inability of the brain and nervous system
generally to adapt themselves to the conditions
which are necessary for sleep. We meet with
this disorder more in private than in hospital
practice. It occurs mostly in persons who are
members of what are known as the upper and
upper middle classes. It occurs mostly in persons of high mental endowment and of neurotic
temperament. The malady is of extreme
importance, and, happily, if its causes be under-
stood and judiciously corrected and controlled,
there are few affections which are more within
the sphere of curative therapeutics. I think I
can succeed in showing you how to unravel the
complex causes and discover the successful
treatment of this kind of insomnia.

The causes and the course of particular
instances of intrinsic insomnia present some
striking differences. You must know these
differences, and be ready to recognise them,

for the knowledge of them clears up alike the therapeutics, the successful treatment, and the prognosis of individual cases of the malady. I have found it to be convenient in practice to arrange the different clinical varieties of such insomnia into groups, in which the cause of the affection is the principle of division. These groups I call respectively the *psychic*, the *toxic*, and the *senile*. Let us see how these divisions work out in detail.

The brain in natural sleep is, as we have seen, relatively anæmic. The cerebral arteries, as we have seen, are more filled with blood than during sleep, when the brain is in full waking and working activity. When thought is active, the parts of the brain concerned are living relatively rapidly; they are actively receiving nourishment from the blood, and they are, too, actively ridding themselves of the waste products of their vitality. In sound natural sleep the brain is inactive, excepting those parts of it which are concerned in the processes of organic life. In sleep the blood flows to and through the brain in streams which are smaller and gentler than in the waking state. The cells concerned in thought, volition, and feeling are not expending energy, they are renewing it and storing it—they are resting.

Any cause, however little we may be able to trace the details of its operation, which directly prevents a repose duly deep of a sufficient number of those brain cells which are the organs of conscious thought, will render sleep impossible; relative cerebral hyperæmia is an inseparable consequence of such activity, and such relative cerebral hyperæmia becomes a concurrent, but subordinate, cause of insomnia. Here there is progression through a vicious circle of two terms, in which the impulse of the morbid movement springs from the cerebral cells. So we see that there are causes of insomnia which we may fairly regard as acting primarily in sustaining cerebral activity, and with it, and in consequence of it, relative cerebral hyperæmia, which hyperæmia becomes a contributory cause of the cells keeping awake.

In some other cases of intrinsic insomnia I think we may regard the malady as arising primarily in a perversion of the cerebral blood supply. Any cause which prevents the brain from becoming relatively anæmic in a sufficient degree for sleep will produce sleeplessness. Any ingested agent which sustains cerebral hyperæmia, or any pathological change which impairs sufficiently the contractility of the smaller cerebral arteries, may prevent wholly, or in

part, the occurrence of such a degree and extent
of cerebral anæmia as is required for the pro-
duction of sleep, and without which sleep
cannot be.

So there are causes of insomnia which act
primarily in exciting and in sustaining a
relative cerebral hyperæmia, and with it, and
in consequence of it a cerebral activity which is
wakeful. Here there is again a progression
through a vicious circle of two terms, but one
in which the impulse of the morbid movement
springs from the cerebral blood vessels. In
conscious cerebral activity, which, as we have
seen, is a complex condition of at least dual
causation, in which thought certainly implies
increased blood flow, and increased blood flow
sustains thought, perhaps it may be considered
that we cannot, with strict accuracy, allow
initiative precedence to either of the causes
which are essential to the common result. In
medical reasoning there is little which is so
difficult as tracing effects up to their causes,
and there is little so easy as the invention of
causes for effects. Let this caution make you
wary. Take due pains in practice to analyse
the causation of each particular case of intrinsic
insomnia. When you make such analysis you
will find that in some cases of sleeplessness, as

in the psychic group, undue and protracted
cerebral activity is the primary vice, and that
in others, as in the toxic and senile varieties,
relative cerebral hyperæmia is the initial error,
and wakeful cerebral action its direct consequence.

Our present consideration of our subject
has advanced to a point at which we may usefully illustrate our generalizations with some
sketches of particular instances of intrinsic
insomnia, as they are met with in medical
practice. In a case of psychic insomnia some
sudden emotional shock of a depressing kind,
as grief at the death of a beloved relative, will
sometimes be found to have produced at once
persistent sleeplessness, which sleeplessness will
only yield to carefully directed therapeutic
procedures. Again, prolonged mental strain,
in all its varied phases, is a common cause of
the psychic variety of insomnia. Our patient
may be a student preparing for an examination.
For weeks, in spite of fatigue, he may have
shortened his hours for sleep that he might
lengthen his time for reading; and he may
have been in the habit of keeping himself
awake, when he could have readily fallen
asleep, by drinking strong tea or coffee, or by
smoking tobacco. But he could always go to

sleep at once when he went to bed, and sleep
soundly, until, after some weeks of his abnormal work, with the nearer approach of the
examination bringing increased anxiety as to
the result of the ordeal, he found he began to
sleep badly or almost not to sleep at all. He
grew miserable; he could not remember what
he read; he felt unfit for any exertion; and he
could not face his examination. Or, our patient
may be a young professional man. He has com-
menced practice, or rather to wait for practice,
as a barrister, a solicitor, a physician, or a
surgeon. He begins to find that causes or cases
have not been waiting for his advent; clients
or patients are " few and far between." For a
time he manfully struggles on, his hope and
his health sustaining him; but these at last
yield under the continued pressure of new
disappointments and accumulating anxieties.
He may want money; his friends will give it
to him readily if he will ask for it, but his pride
prevents him. It is not a gift or a loan he
needs; he does not want to beg or to borrow
money; he yearns to earn it. And while he has
been hoping and waiting, and growing sick
with the failure of his expectations, he has
been working early and late in his exacting
studies—perhaps straining his powers in pre-

paration for some higher examination, and, it maybe withal, adding the denial of due sleep and exercise, and so he has been wasting and wearing his psychical and physical energies, in the trust that he might thus so skill himself the more as to secure the longed-for practice. At last he has fairly broken down. He has grown thinner; he looks haggard; he is filled with groundless fears; he is weighed down with the ineffable misery of insomnia; he has headache constantly, and noises in his ears; he thinks his memory is failing; he is dull and listless; he has been lying awake for hours after going to bed, or, waking in the " small hours," he has been unable to sleep again, and when he has slept he has had horrid dreams; and he comes to us for help because he can scarcely sleep at all, and he is possessed by the fear that he is going mad. His misery is urgent; it excludes all other joys and most other pains; it is the unspeakable misery of intrinsic insomnia, the insomnia which hangs on no solacing peg of causal pain. Here we observe particular instances in which acute or continued mental strain is the primary cause of the sleeplessness. Where the shock has been sudden and severe it has been sufficient to rouse a given group of cells into persistent activity, and to produce psychic insomnia suddenly. So produced, the sleeplessness may become a persistent trouble, which yields only to judicious therapeutic procedures. In other cases, and more commonly, the insomnia has only arisen after prolonged mental strain, as that which a student may undergo in over-reading for an examination, as that of continued financial anxiety, or that of arduous and sustained literary composition. Where the shock has been sudden and severe enough, there has resulted a persistent wakeful activity. Where the strain has been less intense, but kept up long, a monotonous group of ideas has been maintained in exhausting recurrence. In either case it would appear that sleeplessness did not occur until there arose from exhaustion partial or complete vasomotor paralysis of the intra-cranial blood vessels; it arose when the arterioles of the brain had no longer that contractility without which sleep is impossible. In these forms of insomnia unnatural excitation of the cerebral cells is probably the initial fault. This point of view, we shall find just now, gives the best working hypothesis for our treatment.

Here I must further direct your attention to the question of the causal association of what is known as the nervous temperament with intrinsic insomnia, and especially with this

psychic variety of the malady. In my experience, the subjects of the psychic variety of
insomnia are mostly men, and almost invariably
men of the temperament which is known in
medicine as the nervous temperament. I
advise you to study temperaments. Their recog-
nition is of much value in diagnosis, in
prognosis, and in therapeutics. A temperament
may be defined as " that individual peculiarity
of physical organisation by which the manner
of acting, feeling, and thinking of every person
is permanently affected," and the nervous temperament is marked by great sensitiveness and
activity of the nervous system.* We have lately
been too ready to ignore temperaments; our
fathers studied them better and regarded them
more than we do. But I shall not go to any
authority for a portrait of the nervous temperament; I shall describe it to you as I judge I
have found it in a physician's practice. I use
the phrase nervous temperament to indicate a
distinct type of outward form, of manner, of
habits, of tendencies, and of personal aptitudes,
physiological and pathological. Temperaments
present their various types most frequently in

---

* A Medical Lexicon. Published by the New Sydenham
Society.

men. Comparatively few women exhibit a well-marked temperament; but when a woman is of the nervous temperament, in her the temperament is mostly very distinct indeed. In frequent instances, two or more of the different kinds of temperament may appear to be blended in one patient; we have a compound of reciprocally modified temperaments.* A man of distinctly nervous temperament has a quick manner; he is nearly always in a hurry; he is apt to talk volubly and to eat quickly; if he do not know us well, he fidgets in his hands, or legs, or face when he is speaking; he talks abruptly, earnestly, and fluently, often splitting up his phrases, or recalling and correcting them, and especially modifying qualifying words, such as adverbs and adjectives, in his anxious desire to express what he conceives to be the finest shades of truth. A man of this temperament is apt to "overdo" everything into which his feelings enter, and his feelings enter prominently into most of his doings. He is apt for hobbies; and he is often a diligent collector of curiosities. When he becomes a

---

* Clinically, the most marked temperaments are those known respectively by the names of bilious, lymphatic, nervous, and sanguineous.

patient, he is harassed about some trivial symptom; he has felt his heart beating, and he thereupon fancies he has some deadly cardiac disease; he thinks his memory is failing, and he forthwith imagines he is going mad. Your elucidation of temperamental details in medical practice will develop your clinical observation and acumen. *Ars medici est in observationibus* is a maxim of our schools which was a favourite one of that excellent clinician and successful physician, the late Sir Andrew Clark, and this proverb of ours is very true in the detection of the signs of the nervous temperament.

A man who has suffered much from intrinsic insomnia becomes the subject of a well-marked group of symptoms, subjective and objective. Most of them are given by certain writers amongst the signs of cerebral hyperæmia. It is probable that they mark a particular variety of exhaustion of the brain, attended by more or less of an abnormal increase of blood in the brain, and accompanied by some general prostration of the bodily powers. These concomitants of insomnia, as I have found them, I now describe to you. The patient has a dull and listless look; his eyes are wanting in vivacity; the upper lids may droop a little, and they may be

slightly swollen. The complexion is sallow.
There is headache; of this there are two kinds,
which either co-exist or occur separately. The
commoner variety of headache is a dull pain
felt over the whole of the vertex, together with
a vague and widespread feeling of oppression
in the head; the other is a sharp, shooting
pain, which comes on suddenly, and usually
in single flashes, and which gives the idea of
a knife being driven through the head from one
temple to the other. Occasionally the patient
feels giddiness momentarily; this may cause a
false step, but it never lasts long enough to
give rise to staggering. The skin of the scalp,
especially near the sagittal suture, may be
tender. There are noises in the ears, in one or
in both, usually of a low-pitched whistling
character. This tinnitus aurium may come on
suddenly, and without apparent cause, as when
the patient is talking quietly, or it may only
arise when the patient's attention is more
closely occupied, as in writing a letter or in
casting up figures. A striking sign in the group
of symptoms we are considering is a slight
impairment of hearing. The patient may be
unaware of it, but those with whom he lives
have noticed that he often asks them to repeat
what they say to him because he could not quite

catch their words. He may also complain of
seeing spots before his eyes—little cobwebby
black lines, *muscœ volitantes*, which come and
go and float about, or, perhaps, bright, bluish,
phosphorescent-like specks, phosphenes, which
seem fixed for a moment, one before each eye,
and which only appear when he first directs his
eyes towards an object. There are usually some
abnormal sensations in the skin; not formica-
tion, such as is apt to arise in organic nervous
disease, but a sharp, transitory, and isolated
prickling, as of the movement of a single pin,
which lasts only for an instant, and affects
either the limbs or the trunk, mostly the former.
There may be a peculiar twitching of muscles.
This is a state of involuntary muscular movement of which I have made original and inde-
pendent observation, and of which I know of
no previous description, either oral or written.
It is not a vibratory tremor, like that of
progressive muscular atrophy, nor is it a contraction of a whole muscle, or of a group of
muscles, such as arises in true convulsion. But,
while the patient is sitting still, a considerable
part of a muscle becomes the subject of rapid
clonic movements, and these are wholly inde-
pendent of his volition. These movements
mostly occur in one of the lower extremities,

and they are rarely sufficient to move the position of the limb; they usually affect the lower part of one vastus internus, and last for about a minute. The patient can feel the movements by attending to the affected part, and he can also feel that the muscle moves by applying his hand to it. In such a case there is often also an unnatural and painful sensitiveness to external impressions. The patient craves for quiet. A bright light troubles him. Noises, the sight of moving objects, touches, as of the hand of a friend upon his shoulder, annoy him. There is not an increased sensitiveness to external impressions, but impressions which are enjoyed or unnoticed in health become irritants.

In the toxic variety of intrinsic insomnia the cause of the sleeplessness acts primarily upon the blood vessels of the brain, giving rise to some degree of arterial hyperæmia. Cerebral vascularity, especially the arterial supply of the cortex of the brain, is maintained at such a height and so long by some poisonous agent that conscious cerebral activity—that is, wakefulness—is an inevitable consequence. Such a poison may be introduced into the body from without, or it may be a product of diseased processes arising within the body itself. Of course,

I use the word " poison " in a restricted sense;
I do not mean something which kills, but only
something which produces abnormal manifestations in the living body. The poisons with
which we have here to do are not lethal poisons,
but milder noxious agents which produce
certain distinct and abnormal manifestations.
Tobacco, alcohol, tea and coffee are the external
poisons which most frequently cause sleeplessness; internal or autogenetic poisons causing
intrinsic insomnia may be found in certain
waste products of tissue metamorphosis which
accumulate in the bodies of gouty persons, or
in the bodies of persons whose kidneys are
inadequate.

Possibly, as our knowledge of auto-intoxication shall increase, some other forms of auto-
intoxication may be found to cause intrinsic
insomnia, and the exact details of the causal
chain may be made out. Clinical experience
has suggested to me that insomnia may sometimes be a neurosis having its origin in toxic
absorptions by the gastro-intestinal mucous
tract. Certainly intrinsic insomnia is found
in practice to come and go with constipation
and the relief of constipation. The explanation
of such association of symptoms may be a toxic
one. The word " copræmia " is coming into

medical use, to signify a kind of poisoning of
the blood by noxious principles derived from
retained fæces. Sallowness of the skin, what
may be called fæcal anæmia, anorexia,
"biliousness," and asthenia mark this condition, and, in some cases, intrinsic insomnia
may be added to its characteristics.

With regard to the smoking of tobacco,
many a man cannot sleep either sufficiently or
soundly simply because he smokes excessively.
Smokers often find by their own experience
that they sleep badly if they smoke more than
their usual quantity of tobacco, or if they smoke
tobacco of a stronger kind than that to which
they are accustomed. So a smoker who suffers
from insomnia may find the cure of his sleeplessness in the restriction of his smoking. He
need not give up, nor shorten, nor change his
work, nor need he change his "surroundings";
if he restrict his smoking, he soon sleeps well.
So also as to snuff-taking in relation to insomnia.
Men of nervous temperament, or men into whose
temperament there enters a distinct and considerable blending of the nervous element, often
smoke tobacco or take snuff largely. The consumption of tobacco by smoking or snuff-
taking stimulates the cerebral circulation. This
stimulation, if pushed to undue limits, induces

cerebral vasomotor debility, with a consequent tendency to persistent conscious thought, and so to wakefulness.

Similarly, too, the drinking of alcoholic beverages causes insomnia. The man who drinks to commencing drunkenness mostly sleeps soundly, if not well. But many a so-called moderate drinker knows that he sleeps badly if he take a little more than his usual quantity of wine, for instance, after dinner, or even his usual quantity of some unusual wine. Alcohol, when it passes from the stomach to the blood, flushes and dilates the smaller blood vessels, especially those of the brain; if such a condition be maintained, sleep is disturbed or wanting. We have all seen clinical examples of the insomnia of delirium tremens: the patient cannot sleep because the lesser arteries of his brain are weakened, perhaps paralysed, by alcohol, and sleepless cerebral activity is the inevitable consequence. Far short of what is usually called alcoholism, we often meet with cases of insomnia in which alcohol alone is the cause of shortened, interrupted, and disturbed sleep. The patient may pride himself upon his moderate use of fermented stimulants, and he may be wholly ignorant of the cause of the sleeplessness for which he consults us. We fail

to find any sufficient psychic cause for his
insomnia; but if we take away or diminish
his wine or his grog, or induce him to consume
it before the evening, we find he soon begins
to sleep well.

Again, the effects of the consumption of
tea and coffee in causing sleeplessness are well
known. This effect is so obvious that patients
usually remedy it for themselves. As you well
know, tea in the form of an infusion and coffee
in the form of an infusion or of a decoction are
used generally in civilised countries as the daily
beverages of the people. Tea leaves contain
an alkaloid which has been called theine, and
coffee seeds contain an alkaloid which has been
called caffeine, and theine and caffeine have
been shown to be identical; both these leaves
and these seeds contain besides certain oily
principles. With regard to tea, what may be
called its physiological action appears to depend
on the joint action of its theine and of the
volatile oil which tea leaves contain. What is
called green tea is produced by drying the fresh
leaves on a heated iron plate until they become
shrivelled; while black tea is manufactured
by placing the leaves in heaps and allowing
them so to lie while they undergo a kind of
fermentation, after which they are dried.

Green tea and black tea are powerful cerebral stimulants, exciting the mental faculties and the cerebral circulation, and tending to prevent sleep. Coffee, too, is a cerebral stimulant and antisoporific. It is sometimes used in medicine for these properties, to counteract the effects of opium and of its derivative narcotics, and of other narcotic poisons. Some people are extremely susceptible to the sleep-preventing effects of tea or of coffee; others, by use, do not feel such effects, even when considerable quantities of those beverages are consumed. In all cases of bad sleeping you should make sure that tea or coffee is not taken to excess, neither near bedtime.

In gouty persons, quite apart from secondary wakefulness caused by their gouty pains, there may be some intrinsic insomnia, of a kind which is probably toxic in its causation. So, also, intrinsic insomnia may afflict a patient whose kidneys are failing, who has renal inadequacy. In such cases it would seem to appear that the accumulation in the blood, in consequence of deficient excretion, of the products of tissue-metamorphosis causes a general restlessness which disposes to insomnia. Insomnia so caused is not severe, and it is rarely complete. There is slumber rather than

sleep. There is restlessness, perhaps some
excessive irritability to certain external impressions, short and broken sleep, and what may
be called superficial sleep, rather than prolonged wakefulness. In this connection I may
remind you that you should observe the tension
of your patient's pulse. A patient may complain that he sleeps very badly, that he lies in
bed awake for some hours and has great diffi-
culty in " getting off " to sleep, that he sleeps
lightly, awakens often, and dreams much. You
may find he has a pulse of increased and high
tension, with accentuation of the aortic second
sound, and with the cardiac first sound
lengthened and muffled, perhaps reduplicated,
at the apex of the heart. In a case of chronic
kidney disease there may be also the physical
signs which mark the characteristic cardiac
hypertrophy which accompanies chronic con-
tracting nephritis, and is an effect of it or a
concurrent effect of a remoter pathological
cause. Insomnia in such cases is likely to be
due to the maintenance of a state of high
tension in the cerebral arteries, the tension
in them not falling sufficiently for prolonged,
deep, and dreamless sleep. In practice you will
find the causation of many of these cases of
insomnia, and you will find sound therapeutic

indications, too, in the signs of the gouty diathesis or in the discovery of albuminuria. Here I must give you a caution, which you may usefully remember in practice, namely, never accept a patient's statement that he is gouty without the establishment by your own observation of facts sufficient for such a diagnosis. Insomnia which is purely nervous may be wrongly attributed to gout, and depletory measures of treatment may be adopted when corroborants are really indicated. The diagnosis of gout is a diagnosis for which patients often have a tender affection, and I am afraid it is a diagnosis which is often erroneously made, and wrongly handed on through a succession of credulous advisers. Do not fall into the frequent error of making a diagnosis of gout because a specimen of your patient's urine which is brought to you shows a deposit which to the naked eye is like unto grains of cayenne pepper, and which deposit is made up of aggregated crystals of uric acid. Such a sediment may be only an innocent result of an acid fermentation, such as frequently arises in urine after its voidance, without any pathological significance whatsoever.

As I have already told you, there is a senile form of intrinsic insomnia. Remember that

senility is a term of which the primary abso-
luteness is largely modified in particular cases
by relative qualifications. Some persons are
senile early, others only later. With much
truth it may be said that a person is not as old
as his years, at least in a pathological sense,
but as old as his arteries. You may perhaps
have observed amongst your friends that an
exaggerated appreciation of the merits and
value of early rising often increases as age
advances. The broken and short sleep of many
old persons is mainly, if not entirely, the result
of senile degeneration of the smaller cerebral
arteries. In such degeneration those blood
vessels are less elastic and less contractile than
in health, and a degenerative weakening of
their walls often leads to their permanent dilatation; the smaller cerebral arteries, so changed
by a pathological process, are physically unable,
by reason of a diminution of their resilience
and of their contractility, to adapt themselves
normally to such a condition of relative arterial
anæmia as is of the essence of healthy sleep.
The tendency of this condition of the blood
vessels of the brain to prevent, to lessen, or to
interrupt sleep is probably to a great extent
counteracted, in many cases, by the cardiac
feebleness which so frequently, and which,

within certain limits, it may be said fortu-
nately, co-exists with senile vascular changes.
When arteries are brittle, cardiac failure,
within certain limits, may be regarded as a
conservative lesion, in the sense that such
failure tends to save from arterial rupture and
the consequences of cerebral hemorrhage.

II.

THE CURE OF INSOMNIA.*

No "rule of thumb" cure.—Hypnotic drugs.—
Risks from hypnotics.—Causal treatment.—
Bromide of potassium.—Cure of anæmia.—
Alcohol.—Carminatives.—Adjuvant remedies.—
Popular remedies.—Rhythmic sleep.—Physical
exercise.—Sunshine.—Monotonous impressions.
— Bedclothes. — Ventilation. — Food. — Cold.—
Toxic insomnia.—Senile insomnia.

THERE is no "rule of thumb" cure for insomnia.
Each case must be separately studied; the
details of its cure can only be decided under
competent medical advice. I will help you all
I can now in this part of our subject; but
many remedial details are only suggested in
practice by the exigencies of particular cases,
and are only developed as the fruit of long
experience in the treatment of persons suffering from sleeplessness. I shall tell you something of the use of hypnotic drugs, and of the
dangers of some of them; I shall try to impress

---

* A Clinical Lecture: published in *The British Medical*
Journal, December 8th, 1900; since revised and extended.

upon you the importance of stopping overwork, when overwork is a cause of insomnia;
and I shall point out to you many hygienic
considerations which bear upon the cure of
insomnia, and some useful therapeutic adju-
vants which I have found helpful to that end
in my practice, and which may suggest to you
many other successful remedial procedures.

In the treatment of insomnia you may find
it necessary to exhibit some of the drugs which
are known to you as hypnotics or soporifics;
these are remedies that induce sleep. When
you have to deal with a case of insomnia do not
assume that you must of necessity give a
hypnotic drug. I advise you rather to assume
that you can cure a given case of insomnia by
understanding its particular causation and by
remedying the same, rather than by attacking
the effect by dosing the patient with some
hypnotic. Prescribe hypnotics only in exceptional cases; only administer such drugs when
you cannot help it. Your experience in practice will enable you to decide, with increasing
precision, when such an exceptional case is
before you. Rely, whenever you can, upon an
intelligent causal treatment of insomnia, com-
bining such treatment with a judicious employment of some of the non-medicinal helpers of

sleep which I am about to describe to you, if such addition to a strictly causal treatment be needed in any particular case. As a rule, the successful treatment of a case of sleeplessness follows from the discovery of its cause. In the severer forms of psychic insomnia, however, it often happens in practice that we must at once secure sleep by the action of some efficient hypnotic. I prefer opium or chloral. By the use alone of one of these drugs we can often quickly cure acute insomnia depending upon some sudden mental shock or strain. You will find that a few nights of sound and sufficient sleep, artificially induced by the exhibition of a reliable hypnotic, will do more than anything else to restore to the brain the power of sleeping without further aid from drugs. Besides chloral hydrate, opium, morphine, and the other soporific derivatives of opium, the chief hypnotic drugs are sulphonal, trional, paraldehyde, amylene hydrate, and the bromides, to which may be added alcohol and affusion of the head with cold water. For details concerning the comparative merits and demerits of chloral hydrate, paraldehyde, amylene hydrate, sulphonal, and trional, I must refer you to the admirable writings of Professor Binz.*

* Lectures on Pharmacology. New Sydenham Society's Translation.

Sir T. Lauder Brunton insists upon a well-recognised and valuable therapeutic consideration, namely, that a combination of hypnotics is sometimes more successful than any of them singly. He recommends a combination of "small quantities, such as 5 or 10 minims, of solution of opium or morphine, with 5 grains of chloral and 10 to 30 of potassium bromide."* These and other hypnotics may be variously combined to meet the indications of each particular case, according to the judgment of a skilful adviser.

Here I must warn you very plainly and very seriously of the risks which attach to the administration of powerful hypnotic drugs. Many human lives are yearly lost as the consequence of the taking by sufferers from insomnia of overdoses of hypnotics. All drugs which produce sleep as a physiological effect, and the relief of insomnia as a therapeutic action, with the exception, perhaps, of the bromides, produce stupor rather than sleep in overdoses, which deepens into the sleep which knows no waking when they are ingested or injected in larger doses still. So never allow a patient to dose himself with hypnotics. Keep the matter

---

* A Text-Book of Pharmacology, &c.

quite within your own secure hands, upon well-
recognised limits of safety. In the less acute
and more chronic forms of psychic insomnia,
where the sleeplessness or wakefulness usually
depends upon prolonged worry or overwork, I
employ chloral or other powerful dormitives
sparingly. They should only be used as temporary remedies, when it is necessary to secure
at once a fair amount of sleep. A patient
should never be allowed to swallow chloral or
any other of the dangerous but valuable hypnotics whenever he feels so disposed, neither
should he apportion their doses for himself;
he can only safely take them under direct
medical control and observation.

Another important point must not escape
from view. It is this: an overworked man or
woman must never be permitted to go on with
his or her overwork and habitually secure sleep
by chloral or by any other hypnotic. In such
a case we must relentlessly aim at preventing
the sleeplessness by removing its cause, instead
of pursuing the illogical and precarious course,
into which often a wilful and impatient
patient would persuade us, of permitting that
cause to continue, and of trusting to counteract
or suppress the resulting insomnia, a trouble-
some effect of that cause, by medicine.

Remember that work which prevents due sleep is dangerous work. When a man cannot sleep because he works his brain too much, we must make as a condition of our help that he stop or greatly lessen his labour. Especially should he abstain from mental work for some hours before going to bed. In many persons the cerebral hyperæmia of severe mental toil does not fall down to the circulatory limits required for healthy sleep for several hours after the cessation of such work. But I advise you to be wisely suspicious in practice as to accepting work as a cause of insomnia. Nature provides that disposition to rest shall follow work. It is mostly worry, not overwork, or it is work under wrong conditions, which makes sleep difficult.

Whatever the cause of the insomnia, a holiday, with complete change of scene and with distinct change of activities, will often do much to cure. Great as is the curative influence of new surroundings and of new outlets for energy, in many cases of psychic insomnia we cannot, however, do without drugs. Potassium bromide is by far the best hypnotic in well-nourished patients, and in the slighter cases generally. It is marvellously powerful in producing nervous calm; it is a direct brain sedative, and quite a safe one. But it must be given properly, and in full doses; after getting into bed, 30 to 60 grains, dissolved in water, should be the dose. Sometimes you may usefully combine with it some drug which will favour the contraction of the weakened cerebral blood vessels. For this indication we may give tincture of ergot or tincture of digitalis, one or both.

In many cases of chronic wakefulness arising from prolonged mental strain, the patient is distinctly anæmic. The insomnia cannot be cured unless the anæmia be cured. The pallor of the patient's face, the lightened tints of his visible mucous surfaces, and his soft and small pulse, declare the condition of his blood. Such a person mostly feels drowsy when he is up and wakeful when he lies down. He needs hæmatinics, of which the best are iron and arsenic, singly or combined. His diet must be generous, containing plenty of fish, meat, and eggs. For such a patient alcohol is often the best hypnotic; its form and dosage need peculiarly precise prescription and careful supervision.

The prescription of alcohol as a remedy in disease is often difficult and sometimes dangerous. To many people a "nightcap" of

toddy is a superfluous, perhaps hurtful, luxury.
It gives, however, perhaps better than anything
else, rest and sleep to the worried brain of
feeble persons whose blood is poor. I find that
alcohol is the best hypnotic in many cases of
chronic psychic insomnia, when the patient is
worried and weakly, sorrowful and anæmic.
We need not exaggerate our responsibility in
the prescription of alcohol; but we should
never forget it. I have been accustomed to
insist that when we use alcohol, in the form of
any of the fluids which contain it, in the treatment of insomnia, we should explain to our
patient the reasons for the employment of the
remedy, and that we should discontinue this
remedy as we discontinue the use of other
drugs, when the conditions which called for
its exhibition shall have disappeared.

I have found in practice that a carminative,
best taken just after the patient be entered into
bed for a night's sleep, is an efficient remedy
in some cases of intrinsic insomnia. Such a
remedy is indicated when a sense of gastro-
intestinal discomfort, often described by a
patient as a feeling of "sinking" in the
stomach, with or without flatulence, appears
in any particular case to prevent sleep. A carminative is a cheering and comforting remedy,

which relieves gastro-intestinal discomfort,
stomach-ache, or belly-ache, disperses and prevents flatulence, and promotes speedily a feeling
of local well-being, and all this so markedly
that its name may be justified either by the
song of joy which it almost inspires or by a
carmen meaning a charm as well as a tune. Oil
of cajuput is a reliable remedy of this kind. In
its action it is a carminative, an antispasmodic,
and a diffusible stimulant. It may be given
in a dose of five drops, or a little less or a
little more, dropped upon a piece of lump
sugar, or crumb of bread. Hot water, as a
beverage, is also a carminative, diffusible
stimulant, and antispasmodic, promotive of
gastro-intestinal peristalsis. I have read that
a well-known English statesman, now living,
cured himself of sleeplessness by drinking a
tumblerful of hot water, "as hot as could be
drunk," before going to bed.

In slighter cases of intrinsic insomnia
some of our dormitives which are milder than
the ordinary hypnotics are useful. We may
now consider these, which may be regarded as
adjuvant remedies, of tried adoption. Many of
these remedies are what may be called popular
remedies, and a remedy, like a person, is not
always the worse for being popular; they are

" understanded of the people," and you should
understand them too, for it is scarcely convenient that you should run risks of being
beaten in your therapeutics of insomnia by a
non-professional prescription of a remedy of
this class. A drachm of the officinal tincture
of hop is a good dormitive. The slumberous
repute of hop attaches to its aroma. King
George the Third, by the advice of his
physician, slept with his head upon a hop
pillow, *pulvinar lupuli*, a pillow stuffed with
newly-dried hop catkins. It is recorded that
such a pillow was used successfully by our
present King in his severe enteric fever in 1871.
Dr. Berkeley, Lord Bishop of Cloyne, records :
" I have known tar-water procure sleep and
compose the spirits in cruel vigils, occasioned
either by sickness or by too intense application
of the mind."* Tar water, made according to
the formula of this prescribing prelate, is still
to be bought from pharmacists. Amongst
popular remedies for sleeplessness there are :
clove-tea; cowslip wine; nutmeg-tea (nutmeg
may be narcotic in large dose); fennel stalks,
eaten as celery; lettuce, as food, or in some of

* Siris : . . . concerning the virtues of Tar water.
By the Right Rev. Dr. George Berkeley, &c., 2nd Edition.
Dublin, 1744.

its medicinal preparations; onions, as food. What may be called the lore of these popular remedies is very interesting; you may pursue it as an instructive diversion, and as one from which you may gather points of use in medical practice.

There are many other matters to which you must give attention in the treatment of chronic psychic insomnia, if you would follow my advice that you should only give hypnotics in exceptional cases, and only when you really cannot obtain a successful result without them. I can now do little more than mention the more important of such details to you.

Some of them you will find useful in some cases, in other cases others. How best to combine them in any given case experience will teach you. Firstly, whether he sleep well or ill, the patient ought from day to day to go to bed and to get up at fixed and regular times. "Lying in bed in the morning" is not a remedy for insomnia. Healthy sleep is a rhythmic act, and rhythmic sleep must be cultivated. The conditions for the periodic recurrence of sleep must be supplied. An afternoon nap for half an hour or so after a meal, with the feet kept warm before a fire, is helpful, and I have found in practice that it conduces to, rather than hinders, better sleeping in bed at night.

Again, daily bodily exercise in the open air, but always short of great fatigue, must be enjoined. What is called carriage exercise is better than no outdoor change at all, but walking is a far better exercise, and cycling better still, and riding on horseback the best of all. A worn and worrying man, habitually wrapt up in an absorbing torture of self-consciousness, exaggerating his subjectivities, and sleeping badly, must perforce come out of himself, and blot out his self-consciousness with the saving graces of objectivities when he mounts a cycle or a horse's back. Gardening, in the open air, not in conservatories nor in hothouses, affords good exercise, and it is very efficient in keeping up objective attention. Dwellers in towns may find good objective employment, of a kind counteractive of insomnia, in various physical exercises and drills, in fencing with foils, and in other similar recreations, all of which you, as medical advisers, must learn to understand in their several details, so that you may prescribe them intelligently to suit the particular needs and aptitudes of individual patients; many may at least copy Archbishop Whately, who remedied the strain of his logic by splitting his logs, and give their minds a

refreshing and recreative objective bent, and
their muscles healthy work, by cutting up fire-
wood. As to sunshine, we healers welcome the
present therapeutic worship of the sun. Certainly sunshine is a natural tonic and calmative.
In practice you may be sure you will find free
and long daily exposure to sunshine a valuable
adjuvant in the cure of insomnia.

Again, many people have acquired more
or less insomnia in the acquisition of the bad
habit of thinking out their affairs upon getting
into bed. Some patients pursue this bad practice for years, and they often conceal it or
disregard it when they seek medical help for
sleeplessness. In such a case you must find
out this bad habit, and break your patient of
it, for the cure of insomnia. Evoke the
patient's self-control in this regard. In such
cases especially, and in the cure of insomnia
generally, people who find it difficult to get
off to sleep have been advised to count
monotonously, one, two, three, up to a
thousand or more, until they fall asleep; to
picture some familiar scene and keep the mind
fixed upon it; to repeat the letters of the
alphabet over and over again. The late Dr.
Pereira gave some interesting illustrations of
the well-known fact that a continued repetition

of monotonous impressions on the senses of hearing, seeing, or touch, are provocative of sleep. One passage from his monumental work on remedies I may quote to you. Speaking of monotonous impressions in the therapeutics of insomnia, he wrote: " This is the principle of ' the method of procuring sound and refreshing slumber at will ' recommended by the late Mr. Gardner, who called himself the hypnologist. His method was for some time kept secret, and was first made public by Dr. Binns. It is as follows: Let the patient ' turn on his right side, place his head comfortably on the pillow, so that it exactly occupies the angle a line drawn from the head to the shoulder would form, and then, slightly closing the lips, take rather a full inspiration, breathing as much as he possibly can through the nostrils. This, however, is not absolutely necessary, as some persons always breathe through their mouths during sleep, and rest as sound as those who do not. Having taken a full inspiration, the lungs are then to be left to their own action; that is, the respiration is neither to be accelerated nor retarded too much; but a very full inspiration must be taken. The attention must now be fixed upon the action in which the patient is engaged. He must depict to himself that he sees the breath passing from his nostrils in a continuous stream, and the very instant he brings his mind to conceive this apart from all other ideas,' he sleeps. ' The instant the mind is brought to the contemplation of a single sensation, that instant the sensorium abdicates the throne, and the hypnotic faculty steeps it in oblivion.' "*

These various methods seem to be devices for changing the current of conscious cerebration. Amongst my patients I have found the plan of taking deep inspirations commended by many of them. But for the most part these expedients succeed for a night or two only, and they can scarcely be relied upon either exclusively or long. These sundry practices may even keep up wakefulness; when the mind attends to them too closely, they may sustain the self-consciousness which keeps the brain from slipping into slumber. To try hard to go to sleep is often the surest way to keep awake. We do many things best when we forget ourselves, and going to sleep is no exception to the rule.

Again, to promote the sleep of a person in bed, you should make sure that the bedclothes which cover him are sufficient and not

---

* Elements of Materia Medica.

excessive. If the covering bedclothes be
especially arranged in quantity each night by
thermometric guidance, according to the temperature of the air in the patient's bedroom,
so as to secure that the thickness of the upper
bedclothes will give to the occupant of the bed
a general feeling of sleep-inducing and sleep-
sustaining comfort, and not of sleep-preventing discomfort, either from local or from
general chilliness or from local or from general
over-heating, sleep will be powerfully promoted.
And, further, if such arrangements be made
with the knowledge and with the interested
approval of the patient, or by himself, we gain
the valuable adjuvant of his self-confidence as
to his sleeping well, and establish in his mind
for the particular night before him a happy
expectation which is likely to be realised. For
your guidance as to the details of practice
arising from this indication of treatment, I
may tell you that, from observations I have
made, I have found that in a large bedroom
in the middle of a large house, with a window
of the room always kept open, a Fahrenheit
thermometer indicated a temperature of 70°,
or upwards, in the hottest weather, and of 40°,
or less, in the coldest weather, in the country,
at an elevation of about 300 feet above the

sea-level, in mid-England. At a temperature
of 44°, the upper bedclothing should consist
of a sheet, three blankets, a light counterpane,
and a light small blanket, this last not " turned
over " at the upper edge of the bedclothing and
not " turned in at the bottom "; at a temperature of 70°, it should be a sheet only. Between
these extremes of temperature the changes in
the thickness of the covering bedclothes should
be gradual. These extremes should be the ends
of a series of gradations passing through about
nine terms. With a little care you can make a
serviceable thermometric register, marking the
suitable bedclothing for a given external temperature of the bedroom in any particular case,
and so you may cure intrinsic insomnia, and
prevent its recurrence.

In all cases, the bedroom window should
be open all night and all the year round, and
aranged so that it may be so without draught.
The head of the bed should be away from a wall.
The best bed on which to lie is a hair mattress,
covered with a sheet and a blanket, and sup-
ported upon a chain stretcher.

In some cases a little food taken just at
the time for sleeping is an efficient soporific.
You may often observe that the good effects of
a little nourishment—a cup of cocoa or a small

piece of dry bread, taken upon getting into bed
or upon awakening after a slumber which is
too short for a night's rest, are most happy.

You may usefully remember that sleep
may often be induced by the temporary application of cold to the head or to the general
surface of the body. A person who has been
lying awake will often fall asleep at once upon
regaining his bed after getting out of bed and
sousing his head, neck, and hands in cold
water, or after following Charles Dickens's plan
of standing at his bedside until he feels chilly,
and thereupon shaking up and cooling his pil-
lows and bedclothes, and then getting into bed.

In the toxic kinds of insomnia we must
especially endeavour, as I have already suggested to you, to act upon the maxim, " *Cessante
causâ cessat et effectus.*" We must stop or lessen
the consumption of tobacco, alcohol, tea, etc.,
as the case may be. The sufferer from toxic
insomnia will ask you what must be done for
sleep. This is not quite the question; the
question is not what the patient must do, but
rather what the patient must not do. The consumption of something must be left off. When
you have found out the what and when of that
something, the patient's self-control, loyal co-
öperation, and obedience to your directions are

essential to your curing the case. A discussion
of the treatment of gouty insomnia, and of the
sleeplessness arising in some chronic kidney
diseases, would involve a consideration of the
whole question of the therapeutics of the
maladies upon which these forms of wakefulness depend. If you find evidence of copræmia
in a case of insomnia, you must, in any case,
treat the underlying fæcal retention. Such
fæcal retention may be the whole cause, or an
active part of the cause, of the insomnia. Senile
insomnia is very obstinate. Perhaps in the
bromides, with full doses of hop or henbane,
we have the most efficient and least harmful
medicinal means of relief; while the promotion
of sleep may be accomplished by an intelligent
combination of some of the non-medicinal
measures to which I have referred.

Now I must close our consideration of this
interesting subject of the therapeutics of
intrinsic insomnia. I have sketched broad out-
lines for your guidance, which will suggest
to you many other details in your practice.
That the best physician is the physician who is
the best inspirer of hope, Coleridge it was, I
think, who so declared. He was largely right.
Of course, truthful hope. Certainly is this
largely true in nervous maladies. In the cure

of intrinsic insomnia, especially, the best physician is one who is a master of his art and withal the most ingenious inspirer of his patient's desire of cure and belief that it is obtainable.

BY THE SAME AUTHOR.

Just Ready.—Fourth Edition, price 3s. net, 1904, with many
revisions and additions, 8vo., cloth.

Contributions to Practical Medicine.

CONTENTS.—Causes and Cure of Insomnia ; Cure of Gastral-
gia ; Inspection in Diseases of Lungs and Pleuræ ; Accentuation
of the Pulmonary Second Sound of the Heart ; Floating Kidney ;
Cure of Habitual Constipation ; Treatment of Severer Forms of
Constipation ; Intestinal Obstruction ; A form of Backache ;
Unguentum Ranunculi Ficariæ in Hæmorrhoids ; Cure of Ec-
zema ; Cure of Chorea by Arsenic ; Chloride of Calcium in the
Treatment of Pulmonary Tuberculosis ; Medicated Lozenges ;
Fuming Inhalations in Asthma ; Ethereal Tincture of Capsicum ;
Ether in Medication by the Skin ; Diet in Diabetes.

PRESS NOTICES.

"Reminds us of the clinical lectures of the immortal Graves."--*Practitioner.*
"A useful contribution to practical medicine."—*British Med. Journ.*
"Lucidly and agreeably written, and conveying much practical information."
—*Lancet.*
"We cordially commend it to our readers."—*Chemist and Druggist.*
"Typical studies in the English clinical vein."—*New York Med. News.*
"Very nice and instructive reading."—*Brit. and Colonial Druggist.*
"Every sentence which it contains is of value."—*Dublin Journ. Med. Sciences.*
"Its practical contributions are appreciated in the profession."—*Medical Press.*
"Many useful points."—*Merck's Archives* (New York).
"Eminently practical "—*New York Med. Record.*
"Very practical."—*Canadian Journ. Medicine and Surgery.*
"Full of practical points."—*Brooklyn Med. Journ.*
"A valuable addition to the library of the medical practitioner."—*Pharma-
ceutical Journ.*
"Will be read with satisfaction and utility."—*Il Policlinico* (Rome).
"The author . . . hits his mark."—*Midland Med. Journ.*
"A really original book."—*Medicinische Blätter* (Vienna).
"Improvements in the methods of treating various diseases and morbid con-
ditions."—*Med. Bulletin* (Philadelphia).
" . . . a pleasure to read. Good common sense, a wide clinical experi-
ence, and good English . . ."—*St. Thomas's Hosp. Gaz.*
"In a very readable manner gives the result of much clinical study and ex-
perience."—*New Zealand Med. Journ.*
"Always good and sound."—*Austral. Med. Gaz.*
"Contain sound practical hints, of which we fully acknowledge the value."—
Birmingham Med. Rev.
"Copious clinical experience and deeply keen observation are giving their
opinion."—*Schmidt's Jahrbücher der Med*
"A work of decidedly practical value." - *Canadian Druggist.*
"A valuable work from which we might learn much."—*Med. World* (Phila-
delphia).
"Abounds in helpful suggestions "—*Wisconsin Med. Recorder.*
"Will be read with pleasure and profit."—*Quart. Med. Journ.* (Yorkshire).
"Written in an interesting manner, and there is much useful information in
the book."—*Med. Chron.* (Manchester).
"An elegant volume . . we congratulate the author."—*Criterio Cat. Cien.
Med.* (Barcelona).
"So good as to be unequalled."—*Centralbl. Inn. Med.*

BIRMINGHAM : CORNISH BROS.

BY THE SAME AUTHOR.

8VO., CLOTH, WITH THREE PLATES, PP. 251, 1870.

A GUIDE

TO THE

Physical Diagnosis of Diseases

OF THE

Lungs and Heart;

TOGETHER WITH AN INTRODUCTION TO THE EXAMINATION OF
THE URINE.

PRESS NOTICES.

"A digest of the best known facts respecting its subject matter. It conveys instruction in those facts in a lucid manner, and will no doubt be appreciated by many students."—*Brit. and For. Medico-Chirurg. Rev.*

"Full of very good and very instructive material."—*Lancet.*

"An excellent and judicious collection of facts, done by a man who knows his work."—*Medical Times and Gaz.*

8VO., CLOTH, PP. 129, 1889.

Notes on Medical Education,

THREE ESSAYS FOUNDED UPON THREE ADDRESSES DELIVERED
TO MEDICAL STUDENTS.

PRESS NOTICES.

" . . . excellent for medical students . . . displaying much good feeling and considerable literary knowledge."—*Saturday Rev.*

"An admirable little manual, cram full of good advice."—*Midland Counties Herald.*